Keto Chaffle Recipes Cookbook:

A complete cookbook with 50+ tasty and flavorful recipes. Lose weight and lower blood pressure in a few steps

SARAH BUCKLEY

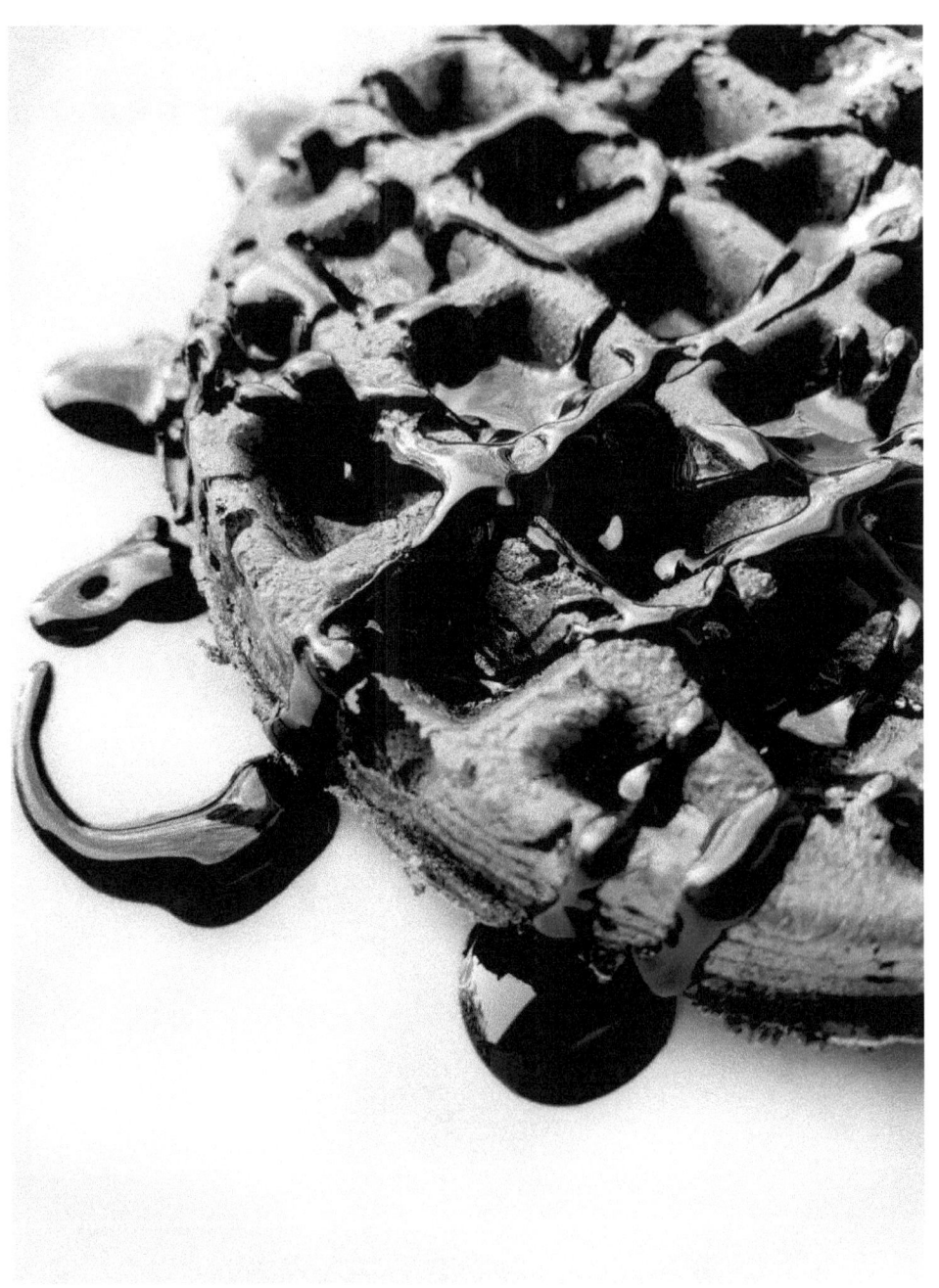

Legal & Disclaimer

The information contained in this book and its contents is not designed to replace or take the place of any form of medical or professional advice; and is not meant to replace the need for independent medical, financial, legal or other professional advice or services, as may be required. The content and information in this book have been provided for educational and entertainment purposes only.

The content and information contained in this book have been compiled from sources deemed reliable, and it is accurate to the best of the Author's knowledge, information, and belief. However, the author cannot guarantee its accuracy and validity and cannot be held liable for any errors and/or omissions. Further, changes are periodically made to this book as and when needed. Where appropriate and/or necessary, you must consult a professional (including but not limited to your doctor, attorney, financial advisor or such other professional advisor) before using any of the suggested remedies, techniques, or information in this book.

Upon using the contents and information contained in this book, you agree to hold harmless the Author from and against any damages, costs, and expenses, including any legal fees potentially resulting from the application of any of the information provided by this book. This disclaimer applies to any loss, damages or injury caused by the use and application, whether directly or indirectly, of any advice or information presented, whether for breach of contract, tort, negligence, personal injury, criminal intent, or under any other cause of action.

You agree to accept all risks of using the information presented inside this book.

You agree that by continuing to read this book, where appropriate and/or necessary, you shall consult a professional (including but not limited to your doctor, attorney, or financial advisor or such other advisor as needed) before using any of the suggested remedies, techniques, or information in this book.

TABLE OF CONTENTS

INTRODUCTION

Whether you want to lose weight or need to burn fat, you can use keve chavel in your diet plan. Keto muffins are a dietary supplement and contain no calories or carbohydrates. It contains low carbohydrates and low calories. Keto foil cakes can help reduce weight.

How it works: The foil skin consists of chopped coconut and pumpkin seeds. It works by providing a low-calorie carbohydrate source that provides energy to your body while keeping blood sugar stable. As you continue to use metal foil, it helps suppress hunger and increase fat burning.

Usually, keto diet therapists will look for precise dietary methods and also find ways to make life easier.

Muffins are one of the foods that stimulate the low-carbohydrate lifestyle. I find them very easy to fix, and thankfully, they can be enjoyed at different times of the day. In the recipe below, I share a variety of ways to make and use muffins-from breakfast to dinner, snacks and desserts.

Therefore, since chaff is rich in healthy fats and most of them are free of carbohydrates, this blending makes dieting easier. Achieving ketosis has become easier!

Finally, they are very convenient to eat. Moreover, we know how preparing meals can help an effective keto diet. Muffins can be frozen for later use, and taste great when heated.

Once you are obsessed with muffins, they will become a key part of your eating due to the benefits they bring.

How to Make Chaffles?

Equipment and Ingredients Discussed

Making chaffles requires five simple steps and nothing more than a waffle maker for flat chaffles and a waffle bowl maker for chaffle bowls.

To make chaffles, you will need two necessary ingredients – eggs and cheese. My preferred cheeses are cheddar cheese or mozzarella cheese. These melt quickly, making them the go-to for most recipes. Meanwhile, always ensure that your cheeses are finely grated or thinly sliced for use.

Now, to make a standard chaffle:

- First, preheat your waffle maker until adequately hot.

- Meanwhile, in a bowl, mix the egg with cheese on hand until well combined.

- Open the iron, pour in a quarter or half of the mixture, and close.

- Cook the chaffle for 5 to 7 minutes or until it is crispy.

- Transfer the chaffle to a plate and allow cooling before serving.

11 Tips to Make Chaffles

My surefire ways to turn out the crispiest of chaffles:

- **Preheat Well:** Yes! It sounds obvious to preheat the waffle iron before usage. However, preheating the iron moderately will not get your chaffles as crispy as you will like. The best way to preheat before cooking is to ensure that the iron is very hot.

- **Not-So-Cheesy:** Will you prefer to have your chaffles less cheesy? Then, use mozzarella cheese.

- **Not-So Eggy**: If you aren't comfortable with the smell of eggs in your chaffles, try using egg whites instead of egg yolks or whole eggs.

- **To Shred or to Slice:** Many recipes call for shredded cheese when making chaffles, but I find sliced cheeses to offer crispier pieces. While I stick with mostly shredded cheese for convenience's sake, be at ease to use sliced cheese in the same quantity. When using sliced cheeses, arrange two to four pieces in the waffle iron, top with the beaten eggs, and some slices of the cheese. Cover and cook until crispy.

- **Shallower Irons:** For better crisps on your chaffles, use shallower waffle irons as they cook easier and faster.

- **Layering:** Don't fill up the waffle iron with too much batter. Work between a quarter and a half cup of total ingredients per batch for correctly done chaffles.

- **Patience:** It is a virtue even when making chaffles. For the best results, allow the chaffles to sit in the iron for 5 to 7 minutes before serving.

- **No Peeking:** 7 minutes isn't too much of a time to wait for the outcome of your chaffles, in my opinion. Opening the iron and checking on the chaffle before it is done stands you a worse chance of ruining it.

- **Crispy Cooling:** For better crisp, I find that allowing the chaffles to cool further after they are transferred to a plate aids a lot.

- **Easy Cleaning:** For the best cleanup, wet a paper towel and wipe the inner parts of the iron clean while still warm. Kindly note that the iron should be warm but not hot!

- **Brush It:** Also, use a clean toothbrush to clean between the iron's teeth for a thorough cleanup. You may also use a dry, rough sponge to clean the iron while it is still warm

SWEET CHAFFLES

1. Cinnamon Swirl Chaffles

Servings: 3

Cooking Time: 12 Minutes

Ingredients:

- For Chaffles:
- 1 organic egg
- ½ cup Mozzarella cheese, shredded
- 1 tablespoon almond flour
- ¼ teaspoon organic baking powder
- 1 teaspoon granulated Erythritol
- 1 teaspoon ground cinnamon
- For Topping:
- 1 tablespoon butter
- 1 teaspoon ground cinnamon
- 2 teaspoons powdered Erythritol

Directions:

1. Preheat a waffle iron and then grease it.

2. For chaffles: in a bowl, place all ingredients and mix until well combined.

3. For topping: in a small microwave-safe bowl, place all ingredients and microwave for about 15 seconds.

4. Remove from microwave and mix well.

5. Place 1/3 of the chaffles mixture into preheated waffle iron.

6. Top with 1/3 of the butter mixture and with a skewer, gently swirl into the chaffles mixture.

7. Cook for about 3-4 minutes or until golden brown.

8. Repeat with the remaining chaffles and topping mixture.

9. Serve warm.

Nutrition: Calories: 87Net Carb: 1gFat: 7.4gSaturated Fat: 3.5gCarbohydrates: 2.1gDietary Fiber: 1.1g Sugar: 0.2gProtein: 3.3g

2. Chocolate Cream Cheese Chaffles

Preparation time: 5 minutes

Cooking Time: 8 Minutes

Servings: 2

Ingredients:

- 1 large organic egg, beaten
- 1 ounce cream cheese, softened
- 1 tablespoon sugar-free chocolate syrup
- 1 tablespoon Erythritol
- ½ tablespoon cacao powder
- ¼ teaspoon organic baking powder
- ½ teaspoon organic vanilla extract

Directions:

1. Preheat a mini waffle iron and then grease it.
2. In a medium bowl, place all ingredients and with a fork, mix until well combined.
3. Place half of the mixture into preheated waffle iron and cook for about 4 minutes or until golden brown.
4. Repeat with the remaining mixture.
5. Serve warm.

Nutrition: Calories: 103Net Carb: 4.2gFat: 7.7gSaturated Fat: 4.1gCarbohydrates: 4.Dietary Fiber: 0.4g Sugar: 2gProtein: 4.5g

3. Colby Jack Chaffles

Servings: 1

Cooking Time: 6 Minutes

Ingredients:

- 2 ounces colby jack cheese, sliced thinly in triangles
- 1 large organic egg, beaten

Directions:

1. Preheat a waffle iron and then grease it.
2. Arrange 1 thin layer of cheese slices in the bottom of preheated waffle iron.
3. Place the beaten egg on top of the cheese.
4. Now, arrange another layer of cheese slices on top to cover evenly.
5. Cook for about 6 minutes.
6. Serve warm.

Nutrition: Calories 292 Net Carbs 2.4 g Total Fat 23 g Saturated Fat 13.6 g Cholesterol 236 mg Sodium 431 mg Total Carbs 2.4 g Fiber 0 g Sugar 0.4 g Protein 18.3 g

4. Chaffle Birthday Cake

Preparation time: 8 minutes

Cooking Time: 16 Minutes

Servings: 2

Ingredients:

- Butter cream icing
- Birthday Cake Chaffle:
- 3 tbsp cream cheese
- 1 tbsp almond flour
- 5 tbsp coconut flour
- 1 tsp baking powder
- 6 eggs
- 2 tbsp birthday cake syrup

Directions:

7. Scoop 3 tbsp of the mixture into your waffle maker. Cook for 4 minutes and set aside.
8. Repeat the process until you have 4 cake chaffles.
9. Just like a normal cake, start assembling your cake by placing one chaffle at the bottom as the base and add a butter cream icing layer. Repeat the same process.

10. Pipe your cake edges with the icing and pile colorful shredded coconut at the center.

11. Once all the layers are completed, top with more icing and shredded coconut sprinkles.

12. Enjoy!

Nutrition: Calories per Servings: 390 Kcal ; Fats: 35 g ;

Carbs: 18.9 g ; Protein: 11 g

5. Chaffle Churros

Preparation time: 5 minutes

Cooking Time: 5 Minutes

Servings: 2

Ingredients:

- 1 egg
- 1 Tbsp almond flour
- ½ tsp vanilla extract
- 1 tsp cinnamon, divided
- ¼ tsp baking powder
- ½ cup shredded mozzarella
- 1 Tbsp swerve confectioners' sugar substitute
- 1 Tbsp swerve brown sugar substitute
- 1 Tbsp butter, melted

Directions:

1. Turn on waffle maker to heat and oil it with cooking spray.
2. Mix egg, flour, vanilla extract, ½ tsp cinnamon, baking powder, mozzarella, and sugar substitute in a bowl.
3. Place half of the mixture into waffle maker and cook for 5 minutes, or until desired doneness.

4. Remove and place the second half of the batter into the maker.
5. Cut chaffles into strips.
6. Place strips in a bowl and cover with melted butter.
7. Mix brown sugar substitute and the remaining cinnamon in a bowl.
8. Pour sugar mixture over the strips and toss to coat them well.

Nutrition: Carbs: 5 g ;Fat: 6 g ;Protein: 5 g ;Calories: 76

6. Strawberry Chaffles

Preparation time: 5 minutes

Cooking Time: 8 Minutes

Servings: 2

Ingredients:

- 1 organic egg, beaten
- ¼ cup Mozzarella cheese, shredded
- 1 tablespoon cream cheese, softened
- ¼ teaspoon organic baking powder
- 1 teaspoon organic strawberry extract
- 2 fresh strawberries, hulled and sliced

Directions:

1. Preheat a mini waffle iron and then grease it.
2. In a bowl, place all ingredients except strawberry slices and beat until well combined.
3. Fold in the strawberry slices.
4. Place half of the mixture into preheated waffle iron and cook for about minutes or until golden brown.
5. Repeat with the remaining mixture.
6. Serve warm.

Nutrition: Calories: 69Net Carb: 1.6gFat: 4.6gSaturated Fat: 2.2gCarbohydrates: 1.9gDietary Fiber: 0.3g Sugar: 1gProtein: 4.2g

7. Butter & Cream Cheese Chaffles

Preparation time: 8 minutes

Cooking Time: 16 Minutes

Servings: 2

Ingredients:

- 2 tablespoons butter, melted and cooled
- 2 large organic eggs
- 2 ounces cream cheese, softened
- ¼ cup powdered erythritol
- 1½ teaspoons organic vanilla extract
- Pinch of salt
- ¼ cup almond flour
- 2 tablespoons coconut flour
- 1 teaspoon organic baking powder

Directions:

1. Preheat a mini waffle iron and then grease it.
2. In a bowl, add the butter and eggs and beat until creamy.
3. Add the cream cheese, erythritol, vanilla extract, and salt, and beat until well combined.

4. Add the flours and baking powder and beat until well combined.

5. Place ¼ of the mixture into preheated waffle iron and cook for about 4 minutes.

6. Repeat with the remaining mixture.

7. Serve warm.

Nutrition: Calories 217   Net Carbs 3.3 g Total Fat 1g Saturated Fat 8.8 g   Cholesterol 124 mg   Sodium 173 mg Total Carbs 6.6 g Fiber 3.3 g Sugar 1.2 g Protein 5.3 g

8. Cinnamon Chaffles

Preparation time: 5 minutes

Cooking Time: 8 Minutes

Servings: 2

Ingredients:

- 1 large organic egg, beaten
- ¾ cup mozzarella cheese, shredded
- ½ tablespoon unsalted butter, melted
- 2 tablespoons blanched almond flour
- 2 tablespoons erythritol
- ½ teaspoon ground cinnamon
- ½ teaspoon Psyllium husk powder
- ¼ teaspoon organic baking powder
- ½ teaspoon organic vanilla extract
- Topping
- 1 teaspoon powdered Erythritol
- ¾ teaspoon ground cinnamon

Directions:

1. Preheat a waffle iron and then grease it.
2. For chaffles: In a medium bowl, put all ingredients and with a fork, mix until well combined.

3. Place half of the mixture into preheated waffle iron and cook for about 5 minutes.
4. Repeat with the remaining mixture.
5. Meanwhile, for topping: in a small bowl, mix together the erythritol and cinnamon.
6. Place the chaffles onto serving plates and set aside to cool slightly.
7. Sprinkle with the cinnamon mixture and serve immediately.

Nutrition: Calories 142 Net Carbs 2.1 g Total Fat 10.6 g Saturated Fat 4 g Cholesterol 106 mg Sodium 122 mg Total Carbs 4.1 g Fiber 2 g Sugar 0.3 g Protein 7.7 g

9. Glazed Chaffles

Preparation time: 5 minutes

Cooking Time: 5 Minutes

Servings: 2

Ingredients:

- ½ cup mozzarella shredded cheese
- ⅛ cup cream cheese
- 2 Tbsp unflavored whey protein isolate
- 2 Tbsp swerve confectioners' sugar substitute
- ½ tsp baking powder
- ½ tsp vanilla extract
- 1 egg
- For the glaze topping:
- 2 Tbsp heavy whipping cream
- 3-4 Tbsp swerve confectioners' sugar substitute
- ½ tsp vanilla extract

Directions:

1. Turn on waffle maker to heat and oil it with cooking spray.

2. In a microwave-safe bowl, mix mozzarella and cream cheese. Heat at 30 second intervals until melted and fully combined.

3. Add protein, 2 Tbsp sweetener, baking powder to cheese. Knead with hands until well incorporated.

4. Place dough into a mixing bowl and beat in egg and vanilla until a smooth batter forms.

5. Put ⅓ of the batter into waffle maker, and cook for 3-minutes, until golden brown.

6. Repeat until all 3 chaffles are made.

7. Beat glaze ingredients in a bowl and pour over chaffles before serving.

Nutrition: Carbs: 4 g ;Fat: 6 g ;Protein: 4 g ;Calories: 130

10. <u>Blueberry Cream Cheese Chaffles</u>

Preparation time: 5 minutes

Cooking Time: 8 Minutes

Servings: 2

Ingredients:

- 1 organic egg, beaten
- 1 tablespoon cream cheese, softened
- 3 tablespoons almond flour
- ¼ teaspoon organic baking powder
- 1 teaspoon organic blueberry extract
- 5-6 fresh blueberries

Directions:

1. Preheat a mini waffle iron and then grease it.
2. In a bowl, place all the ingredients except blueberries and beat until well combined.
3. Fold in the blueberries.
4. Divide the mixture into 5 portions.
5. Place 1 portion of the mixture into preheated waffle iron and cook for about 3-4 minutes or until golden brown.
6. Repeat with the remaining mixture.

7. Serve warm.

Nutrition: Calories: 120Net Carb: 1.Fat: 9.6gSaturated Fat: 2.2gCarbohydrates: 3.1gDietary Fiber: 1.3g Sugar: 1gProtein: 3.2g

SAVORY CHAFFLES RECIPES

11. Herb Chaffles

Preparation time: 10 minutes

Cooking Time: 12 Minutes

Servings: 2

Ingredients:

- 4 tablespoons almond flour
- 1 tablespoon coconut flour
- 1 teaspoon mixed dried herbs
- ½ teaspoon organic baking powder
- ¼ teaspoon garlic powder
- ¼ teaspoon onion powder
- Salt and ground black pepper, to taste
- ¼ cup cream cheese, softened
- 3 large organic eggs
- ½ cup cheddar cheese, grated
- 1/3 cup Parmesan cheese, grated

Directions:

1. Preheat a waffle iron and then grease it.

2. In a bowl, mix together the flours, dried herbs, baking powder, and seasoning, and mix well.

3. In a separate bowl, put cream cheese and eggs and beat until well combined.

4. Add the flour mixture, cheddar, and Parmesan cheese, and mix until well combined.

5. Place the desired amount of the mixture into preheated waffle iron and cook for about 2–3 minutes.

6. Repeat with the remaining mixture.

7. Serve warm.

Nutrition: Calories 240   Net Carb: g Total Fat 19 g Saturated Fat 5 g Cholesterol 176 mg Sodium 280 mg Total Carbs 4 g Fiber 1.6 g Sugar 0.7 g Protein 12.3 g

12. Scallion Chaffles

Preparation time: 6 minutes

Cooking Time: 8 Minutes

Servings: 2

Ingredients:

- 1 organic egg, beaten
- ½ cup Mozzarella cheese, shredded
- 1 tablespoon scallion, chopped
- ½ teaspoon Italian seasoning

Directions:

1. Preheat a mini waffle iron and then grease it.
2. In a medium bowl, place all ingredients and with a fork, mix until well combined.
3. Place half of the mixture into preheated waffle iron and cook for about 4 minutes or until golden brown.
4. Repeat with the remaining mixture.
5. Serve warm.

Nutrition: Calories: 5et Carb: 0.7gFat: 3.8gSaturated Fat: 1.5gCarbohydrates: 0.8gDietary Fiber: 0.g Sugar: 0.3gProtein: 4.8g

13. <u>Eggs Benedict Chaffle</u>

Preparation time: 6 minutes

Cooking Time: 10 Minutes

Servings: 2

Ingredients:

- For the chaffle:
- 2 egg whites
- 2 Tbsp almond flour
- 1 Tbsp sour cream
- ½ cup mozzarella cheese
- For the hollandaise:
- ½ cup salted butter
- 4 egg yolks
- 2 Tbsp lemon juice
- For the poached eggs:
- 2 eggs
- 1 Tbsp white vinegar
- 3 oz deli ham

Directions:

1. Whip egg white until frothy, then mix in remaining ingredients.

2. Turn on waffle maker to heat and oil it with cooking spray.

3. Cook for 7 minutes until golden brown.

4. Remove chaffle and repeat with remaining batter.

5. Fill half the pot with water and bring to a boil.

6. Place heat-safe bowl on top of pot, ensuring bottom doesn't touch the boiling water.

7. Heat butter to boiling in a microwave.

8. Add yolks to double boiler bowl and bring to boil.

9. Add hot butter to the bowl and whisk briskly. Cook until the egg yolk mixture has thickened.

10. Remove bowl from pot and add in lemon juice. Set aside.

11. Add more water to pot if needed to make the poached eggs (water should completely cover the eggs). Bring to a simmer. Add white vinegar to water.

12. Crack eggs into simmering water and cook for 1 minute 30 seconds. Remove using slotted spoon.

13. Warm chaffles in toaster for 2-3 minutes. Top with ham, poached eggs, and hollandaise sauce.

Nutrition: Carbs: 4 g ;Fat: 26 g ;Protein: 26 g ;Calories: 365

14. Chicken Bacon Chaffle

Preparation time: 6 minutes

Cooking Time: 5 Minutes

Servings: 2

Ingredients:

- 1 egg
- ⅓ cup cooked chicken, diced
- 1 piece of bacon, cooked and crumbled
- ⅓ cup shredded cheddar jack cheese
- 1 tsp powdered ranch dressing

Directions:

1. Turn on waffle maker to heat and oil it with cooking spray.
2. Mix egg, dressing, and Monterey cheese in a small bowl.
3. Add bacon and chicken.
4. Add half of the batter to the waffle maker and cook for 3-minutes.
5. Remove and cook remaining batter to make a second chaffle.
6. Let chaffles sit for 2 minutes before serving.

Nutrition: Carbs: 2 g ;Fat: 14 g ;Protein: 16 g ;Calories: 200

15. **Bacon & Veggies Chaffles**

Servings: 6

Cooking Time: 24 Minutes

Ingredients:

- 2 cooked bacon slices, crumbled
- ½ cup frozen chopped spinach, thawed and squeezed
- ½ cup cauliflower rice
- 2 organic eggs
- ½ cup Cheddar cheese, shredded
- ½ cup Mozzarella cheese, shredded
- ¼ cup Parmesan cheese, grated
- 1 tablespoon butter, melted
- 1 teaspoon garlic powder
- 1 teaspoon onion powder

Directions:

1. Preheat a mini waffle iron and then grease it.
2. In a bowl, place all the ingredients except blueberries and beat until well combined.
3. Fold in the blueberries.
4. Divide the mixture into 6 portions.

5. Place 1 portion of the mixture into preheated waffle iron and cook for about 3-4 minutes or until golden brown.

6. Repeat with the remaining mixture.

7. Serve warm.

Nutrition: Calories: 10et Carb: 1.2gFat: 8.4gSaturated Fat: 4.6gCarbohydrates: 1.5gDietary Fiber: 0.3g Sugar: 0.6gProtein: 7.1g

16. Garlic Cheese Chaffle Bread Sticks

Servings: 8

Cooking Time: 5 Minutes

Ingredients:

- 1 medium egg
- ½ cup mozzarella cheese, grated
- 2 Tbsp almond flour
- ½ tsp garlic powder
- ½ tsp oregano
- ½ tsp salt
- For the toppings:
- 2 Tbsp butter, unsalted softened
- ½ tsp garlic powder
- ¼ cup grated mozzarella cheese
- 2 tsp dried oregano for sprinkling

Directions:

1. Turn on waffle maker to heat and oil it with cooking spray.
2. Beat egg in a bowl.
3. Add mozzarella, garlic powder, flour, oregano, and salt, and mix.

4. Spoon half of the batter into the waffle maker.

5. Close and cook for minutes. Remove cooked chaffle.

6. Repeat with remaining batter.

7. Place chaffles on a tray and preheat the grill.

8. Mix butter with garlic powder and spread over the chaffles.

9. Sprinkle mozzarella over top and cook under the broiler for 2-3 minutes, until cheese has melted.

Nutrition: Carbs: 1 g ;Fat: 7 g ;Protein: 4 g ;Calories: 74

17. Simple Savory Chaffles

Preparation time: 6 minutes

Cooking Time: 8 Minutes

Servings: 4

Ingredients:

- 1 large organic egg, beaten
- ½ cup Cheddar cheese, shredded
- Pinch of salt and freshly ground black pepper

Directions:

1. Preheat a mini waffle iron and then grease it.
2. In a bowl, place all the ingredients and beat until well combined.
3. Place half of the mixture into preheated waffle iron and cook for about 4 minutes or until golden brown.
4. Repeat with the remaining mixture.
5. Serve warm.

Nutrition: Calories: 150Net Carb: 0.Fat: 11.9gSaturated Fat: 6.7gCarbohydrates: 0.6gDietary Fiber: 0g Sugar: 0.3gProtein: 10.2g

18. Parmesan Garlic Chaffle

Preparation time: 6 minutes

Cooking Time: 5 Minutes

Servings: 2

Ingredients:

- 1 Tbsp fresh garlic minced
- 2 Tbsp butter
- 1-oz cream cheese, cubed
- 2 Tbsp almond flour
- 1 tsp baking soda
- 2 large eggs
- 1 tsp dried chives
- ½ cup parmesan cheese, shredded
- ¾ cup mozzarella cheese, shredded

Directions:

1. Heat cream cheese and butter in a saucepan over medium-low until melted.
2. Add garlic and cook, stirring, for minutes.
3. Turn on waffle maker to heat and oil it with cooking spray.

4. In a small mixing bowl, whisk together flour and baking soda, then set aside.

5. In a separate bowl, beat eggs for 1 minute 30 seconds on high, then add in cream cheese mixture and beat for 60 seconds more.

6. Add flour mixture, chives, and cheeses to the bowl and stir well.

7. Add ¼ cup batter to waffle maker.

8. Close and cook for 4 minutes, until golden brown.

9. Repeat for remaining batter.

10. Add favorite toppings and serve.

Nutrition: Carbs: 5 g ;Fat: 33 g ;Protein: 19 g ;Calories: 385

19. Chicken & Veggies Chaffles

Preparation time: 10 minutes

Cooking Time: 15 Minutes

Servings: 2

Ingredients:

- 1/3 cup cooked grass-fed chicken, chopped
- 1/3 cup cooked spinach, chopped
- 1/3 cup marinated artichokes, chopped
- 1 organic egg, beaten
- 1/3 cup Mozzarella cheese, shredded
- 1 ounce cream cheese, softened
- ¼ teaspoon garlic powder

Directions:

1. Preheat a mini waffle iron and then grease it.
2. In a medium bowl, place all ingredients and mix until well combined.
3. Place 1/of the mixture into preheated waffle iron and cook for about 4-5 minutes or until golden brown.
4. Repeat with the remaining mixture.
5. Serve warm.

Nutrition: Calories: 95Net Carb: 1.3gFat: 5.8gSaturated Fat: 1.3gCarbohydrates: 2.2gDietary Fiber: 0.9g Sugar: 0.3gProtein: 8.

20. **Turkey Chaffles**

Preparation time: 10 minutes

Cooking Time: 16 Minutes

Servings: 2

Ingredients:

- ½ cup cooked turkey meat, chopped
- 2 organic eggs, beaten
- ½ cup Parmesan cheese, grated
- ½ cup Mozzarella, shredded
- ¼ teaspoon poultry seasoning
- ¼ teaspoon onion powder

Directions:

1. Preheat a mini waffle iron and then grease it.
2. In a medium bowl, place all ingredients and mix until well combined.
3. Place ¼ of the mixture into preheated waffle iron and cook for about 4 minutes or until golden brown.
4. Repeat with the remaining mixture.
5. Serve warm.

Nutrition: Calories: 108Net Carb: 0.5gFat: 1gSaturated Fat: 2.6gCarbohydrates: 0.5gDietary Fiber: 0g Sugar: 0.2gProtein: 12.9g

CHAFFLE CAKE & SANDWICH RECIPES

21. Tomato Sandwich Chaffles

Preparation time: 6 minutes

Servings: 2

Cooking Time: 6 Minutes

Ingredients:

- Chaffles
- 1 large organic egg, beaten
- ½ cup colby jack cheese, shredded finely
- 1/8 teaspoon organic vanilla extract
- Filling
- 1 small tomato, sliced
- 2 teaspoons fresh basil leaves

Directions:

1. Preheat a mini waffle iron and then grease it.
2. For chaffles: in a small bowl, place all the ingredients and stir to combine.

3. Place half of the mixture into preheated waffle iron and cook for about minutes.

4. Repeat with the remaining mixture.

5. Serve each chaffle with tomato slices and basil leaves.

Nutrition: Calories 155 Net Carbs 2.4 g Total Fat 11.g Saturated Fat 6.8 g Cholesterol 118 mg Sodium 217 mg Total Carbs 3 g Fiber 0.6 g Sugar 1.4 g Protein 9.6 g

22. Chocolate Chaffle Cake

Preparation time: 6 minutes

Servings: 2

Cooking Time: 8 Minutes

Ingredients:

- Chocolate Chaffle Cake Ingredients:
- 2 tablespoons cocoa powder
- 2 tablespoons Swerve granulated sweetener
- 1 egg
- 1 tablespoon heavy whipping cream
- 1 tablespoon almond flour
- 1/4 tsp baking powder
- 1/2 tsp vanilla extract
- Cream Cheese Frosting:
- 2 tablespoons cream cheese
- 2 teaspoons swerve confectioners
- 1/8 tsp vanilla extract
- 1 tsp heavy cream

Directions:

1. How to Make Chocolate Chaffle Cake:

2. In a small bowl, whisk together cocoa powder, swerve, almond flour, and baking powder.

3. Add in the vanilla extract and heavy whipping cream and mix well.

4. Add in the egg and mix well. Be sure to scrape the sides of the bowl to get all of the ingredients mixed well.

5. Let sit for 3-4 minutes while the mini waffle maker heats up.

6. Add half of the waffle mixture to the waffle maker and cook for 4 minutes. Then cook the second waffle. While the second chocolate keto waffle is cooking, make your frosting.

7. How to Make Cream Cheese Frosting:

8. In a small microwave-safe bowl add 2 tablespoons cream cheese. Microwave the cream cheese for seconds to soften the cream cheese.

9. Add in heavy whipping cream and vanilla extract and use a small hand mixer to mix well.

10. Then add in the confectioners swerve and use the hand mixer to incorporate and fluffy the frosting.

11. Assembling Keto Chocolate Chaffle cake:

12. Place one chocolate chaffle on a plate, top with a layer of frosting. You can spread it with a knife or use a pastry bag and pipe the frosting.

13. Put the second chocolate chaffle on top of the frosting layer and then spread or pipe the rest of the frosting on top.

Nutrition: (per serving):Calories: 151kcal ;Carbohydrates:5g ;Protein: 6g;Fat: 13g ;Saturated Fat:6g ;Cholesterol:111mg ;Sodium:83mg ;Potassium: 190mg ;Fiber: 2g ;Sugar: 1g ;Vitamin A: 461IU ;Calcium: 67mg ;Iron: 1mg

23. Salmon & Cream Sandwich Chaffles

Preparation time: 6 minutes

Servings: 2

Cooking Time: 8 Minutes

Ingredients:

- Chaffles
- 1 organic egg, beaten
- ½ cup cheddar cheese, shredded
- 1 tablespoon almond flour
- 1 tablespoon fresh rosemary, chopped
- Filling
- ¼ cup smoked salmon
- 1 teaspoon fresh dill, chopped
- 2 tablespoons cream

Directions:

1. Preheat a mini waffle iron and then grease it.
2. For chaffles: In a medium bowl, put all ingredients and with a fork, mix until well combined. Place half of the mixture into preheated waffle iron and cook for about 3–4 minutes.
3. Repeat with the remaining mixture.

4. Serve each chaffle with filling ingredients.

Nutrition: Calories 202 Net Carbs 1.7 g Total Fat 11 g Saturated Fat 7.5 g Cholesterol 118 mg Sodium 345 mg Total Carbs 2.9 g Fiber 1.2 g Sugar 0.7 g Protein 13.2 g

24. Tuna Sandwich Chaffles

Preparation time: 6 minutes

Servings: 2

Cooking Time: 8 Minutes

Ingredients:

- Chaffles
- 1 organic egg, beaten
- ½ cup cheddar cheese, shredded
- 1 tablespoon almond flour
- Pinch of salt
- Filling
- ¼ cup water-packed tuna, flaked
- 2 lettuce leaves

Directions:

1. Preheat a mini waffle iron and then grease it.
2. For chaffles: In a medium bowl, put all ingredients and with a fork, mix until well combined. Place half of the mixture into preheated waffle iron and cook for about 3–4 minutes.
3. Repeat with the remaining mixture.

4. Serve each chaffle with filling ingredients.

Nutrition: Calories 186 Net Carbs 0.9 g Total Fat 13.6 g Saturated Fat 6.8 g Cholesterol 120 mg Sodium 342 mg Total Carbs 1.3 g Fiber 0.4 g Sugar 0.g Protein 13.6 g

CHAFFLE MEAT RECIPES

25. Italian Chicken and Basil Chaffle

Preparation time: 10 minutes

Cooking Time:7–9 Minutes

Servings: 2

Ingredients:

- Batter
- ½ pound ground chicken
- 4 eggs
- 3 tablespoons tomato sauce
- Salt and pepper to taste
- 1 cup grated mozzarella cheese
- 1 teaspoon dried oregano
- 3 tablespoons freshly chopped basil leaves
- ½ teaspoon dried garlic
- Other
- 2 tablespoons butter to brush the waffle maker
- ¼ cup tomato sauce for serving
- 1 tablespoon freshly chopped basil for serving

Directions:

1. Preheat the waffle maker.
2. Add the ground chicken, eggs and tomato sauce to a bowl and season with salt and pepper.
3. Add the mozzarella cheese and season with dried oregano, freshly chopped basil and dried garlic.
4. Mix until fully combined and batter forms.
5. Brush the heated waffle maker with butter and add a few tablespoons of the chaffle batter.
6. Close the lid and cook for about 7–9 minutes depending on your waffle maker.
7. Repeat with the rest of the batter.
8. Serve with tomato sauce and freshly chopped basil on top.

Nutrition: Calories 250, fat 15.7 g, carbs 2.5 g, sugar 1.5 g, Protein 24.5 g, sodium 334 mg

26. Beef Meatballs on A Chaffle

Preparation time: 10 minutes

Cooking Time:20 Minutes

Servings: 2

Ingredients:

- Batter
- 4 eggs
- 2½ cups grated gouda cheese
- ¼ cup heavy cream
- Salt and pepper to taste
- 1 spring onion, finely chopped
- Beef meatballs
- 1 pound ground beef
- Salt and pepper to taste
- 2 teaspoons Dijon mustard
- 1 spring onion, finely chopped
- 5 tablespoons almond flour
- 2 tablespoons butter
- Other
- 2 tablespoons cooking spray to brush the waffle maker
- 2 tablespoons freshly chopped parsley

Directions:

1. Preheat the waffle maker.
2. Add the eggs, grated gouda cheese, heavy cream, salt and pepper and finely chopped spring onion to a bowl.
3. Mix until combined and batter forms.
4. Brush the heated waffle maker with cooking spray and add a few tablespoons of the batter.
5. Close the lid and cook for about 7 minutes depending on your waffle maker.
6. Meanwhile, mix the ground beef meat, salt and pepper, Dijon mustard, chopped spring onion and almond flour in a large bowl.
7. Form small meatballs with your hands.
8. Heat the butter in a nonstick frying pan and cook the beef meatballs for about 3–4 minutes on each side.
9. Serve each chaffle with a couple of meatballs and some freshly chopped parsley on top.

Nutrition: Calories 670, fat 47.4g, carbs 4.6 g, sugar 1.7 g, Protein 54.9 g, sodium 622 mg

27. Leftover Turkey Chaffle

Preparation time: 10 minutes

Cooking Time:7–9 Minutes

Servings: 2

Ingredients:

- Batter
- ½ pound shredded leftover turkey meat
- 4 eggs
- 1 cup grated provolone cheese
- Salt and pepper to taste
- 1 teaspoon dried basil
- ½ teaspoon dried garlic
- 3 tablespoons sour cream
- 2 tablespoons coconut flour
- Other
- 2 tablespoons cooking spray for greasing the chaffle maker
- ¼ cup cream cheese for serving the chaffles

Directions:

1. Preheat the waffle maker.

2. Add the leftover turkey, eggs and provolone cheese to a bowl and season with salt and pepper, dried basil and dried garlic.

3. Add the sour cream and coconut flour and mix until batter forms.

4. Brush the heated waffle maker with cooking spray and add a few tablespoons of the chaffle batter.

5. Close the lid and cook for about 7–9 minutes depending on your waffle maker.

6. Repeat with the rest of the batter.

7. Serve with cream cheese on top of each chaffle.

Nutrition: Calories 372, fat 27.g, carbs 5.4 g, sugar 0.6 g, Protein 25 g, sodium 795 mg

28. Beef Meatza Chaffle

Preparation time: 10 minutes

Cooking Time:15 Minutes

Servings: 2

Ingredients:

- Meatza chaffle batter
- ½ pound ground beef
- 4 eggs
- 2 cups grated cheddar cheese
- Salt and pepper to taste
- 1 teaspoon Italian seasoning
- 2 tablespoons tomato sauce
- Other
- 2 tablespoons cooking spray to brush the waffle maker
- ¼ cup tomato sauce for serving
- 2 tablespoons freshly chopped basil for serving

Directions:

1. Preheat the waffle maker.
2. Add the ground beef, eggs, grated cheddar cheese, salt and pepper, Italian seasoning and tomato sauce to a bowl.

3. Mix until everything is fully combined.

4. Brush the heated waffle maker with cooking spray and add a few tablespoons of the batter.

5. Close the lid and cook for about 7–10 minutes depending on your waffle maker.

6. Serve with tomato sauce and freshly chopped basil on top.

Nutrition: Calories 4, fat 34.6 g, carbs 2.5 g, sugar 1.7 g, Protein 36.5 g, sodium 581 mg

29. Chicken Jalapeno Chaffle

Preparation time: 10 minutes

Cooking Time:8–10 Minutes

Servings: 2

Ingredients:

- Batter
- ½ pound ground chicken
- 4 eggs
- 1 cup grated mozzarella cheese
- 2 tablespoons sour cream
- 1 green jalapeno, chopped
- Salt and pepper to taste
- 1 teaspoon dried oregano
- ½ teaspoon dried garlic
- Other
- 2 tablespoons butter to brush the waffle maker
- ¼ cup sour cream to garnish
- 1 green jalapeno, diced, to garnish

Directions:

1. Preheat the waffle maker.

2. Add the ground chicken, eggs, mozzarella cheese, sour cream, chopped jalapeno, salt and pepper, dried oregano and dried garlic to a bowl.

3. Mix everything until batter forms.

4. Brush the heated waffle maker with butter and add a few tablespoons of the batter.

5. Close the lid and cook for about 8–10 minutes depending on your waffle maker.

6. Serve with a tablespoon of sour cream and sliced jalapeno on top.

Nutrition: Calories 284, fat 19.4 g, carbs 2.2 g, sugar 0.6 g, Protein 24.g, sodium 204 mg

30. Lamb Chops On Chaffle

Preparation time: 10 minutes

Cooking Time:15 Minutes

Servings: 2

Ingredients:

- 4 eggs
- 2 cups grated mozzarella cheese
- Salt and pepper to taste
- 1 teaspoon garlic powder
- ¼ cup heavy cream
- 6 tablespoons almond flour
- 2 teaspoons baking powder
- Lamb chops
- 2 tablespoons herbed butter
- 1 pound lamb chops
- Salt and pepper to taste
- 1 teaspoon freshly chopped rosemary
- Other
- 2 tablespoons butter to brush the waffle maker
- 2 tablespoons freshly chopped parsley for garnish

Directions:

1. Preheat the waffle maker.
2. Add the eggs, mozzarella cheese, salt and pepper, garlic powder, heavy cream, almond flour and baking powder to a bowl.
3. Mix until combined.
4. Brush the heated waffle maker with butter and add a few tablespoons of the batter.
5. Close the lid and cook for about 7 minutes depending on your waffle maker.
6. Meanwhile, heat a nonstick frying pan and rub the lamb chops with herbed butter, salt and pepper, and freshly chopped rosemary.
7. Cook the lamb chops for about 3–4 minutes on each side.
8. Serve each chaffle with a few lamb chops and sprinkle on some freshly chopped parsley for a nice presentation.

Nutrition: Calories 537, fat 37.3 g, carbs 5.5 g, sugar 0.6 g, Protein 44.3 g, sodium 328 mg

SPECIAL CHAFFLE RECIPES

31. Breakfast festive Chaffle Sandwich

Preparation time: 10 minutes

Cooking Time:10 Minutes

Servings: 2

Ingredients:

- 2 basics cooked chaffles

- Cooking spray

- 2 slices bacon

- 1 egg

Directions:

1. Spray your pan with oil.

2. Place it over medium heat.

3. Cook the bacon until golden and crispy.

4. Put the bacon on top of one chaffle.

5. In the same pan, cook the egg without mixing until the yolk is set.

6. Add the egg on top of the bacon.

7. Top with another chaffle.

Nutrition: Calories 514 Total Fat 47 g Saturated Fat 27 g Cholesterol 274 mg Sodium 565 mg Potassium 106 mg Total Carbohydrate 2 g Dietary Fiber 1 g Protein 21 g Total Sugars 1 g

32. **Cookie Dough Chaffle**

Preparation time: 5 minutes

Cooking Time:7–9 Minutes

Servings: 2

Ingredients:

- Batter
- 4 eggs
- ¼ cup heavy cream
- 1 teaspoon vanilla extract
- ¼ cup stevia
- 6 tablespoons coconut flour
- 1 teaspoon baking powder
- Pinch of salt
- ¼ cup unsweetened chocolate chips
- Other
- 2 tablespoons cooking spray to brush the waffle maker
- ¼ cup heavy cream, whipped

Directions:

1. Preheat the waffle maker.

2. Add the eggs and heavy cream to a bowl and stir in the vanilla extract, stevia, coconut flour, baking powder, and salt. Mix until just combined.

3. Stir in the chocolate chips and combine.

4. Brush the heated waffle maker with cooking spray and add a few tablespoons of the batter.

5. Close the lid and cook for about 7–8 minutes depending on your waffle maker.

6. Serve with whipped cream on top.

Nutrition: Calories 3, fat 32.3 g, carbs 12.6 g, sugar 0.5 g, Protein 9 g, sodium 117 mg

33. **Thanksgiving Pumpkin Spice Chaffle**

Preparation time: 5 minutes

Cooking Time:5minutes

Servings: 2

Ingredients:

- 1 cup egg whites
- ¼ cup pumpkin puree
- 2 tsps. pumpkin pie spice
- 2 tsps. coconut flour
- ½ tsp. vanilla
- 1 tsp. baking powder
- 1 tsp. baking soda
- 1/8 tsp cinnamon powder
- 1 cup mozzarella cheese, grated
- 1/2 tsp. garlic powder

Directions:

1. Switch on your square waffle maker. Spray with non-stick spray.
2. Beat egg whites with beater, until fluffy and white.
3. Add pumpkin puree, pumpkin pie spice, coconut flour in egg whites and beat again.

4. Stir in the cheese, cinnamon powder, garlic powder, baking soda, and powder.

5. Pour ½ of the batter in the waffle maker.

6. Close the maker and cook for about 3 minutes Utes.

7. Repeat with the remaining batter.

8. Remove chaffles from the maker.

9. Serve hot and enjoy!

Nutrition: Protein: 51% 66 kcal Fat: 41% 53 kcal Carbohydrates: 8% kcal

34. **Pumpkin Spice Chaffles**

Preparation time: 10 minutes

Cooking Time: 14 Minutes

Servings: 2

Ingredients:

- 1 egg, beaten
- ½ tsp pumpkin pie spice
- ½ cup finely grated mozzarella cheese
- 1 tbsp sugar-free pumpkin puree

Directions:

1. Preheat the waffle iron.
2. In a medium bowl, mix all the ingredients.
3. Open the iron, pour in half of the batter, close, and cook until crispy, 6 to 7 minutes.
4. Remove the chaffle onto a plate and set aside.
5. Make another chaffle with the remaining batter.
6. Allow cooling and serve afterward.

Nutrition: Calories 90Fats 6.46gCarbs 1.98gNet Carbs 1.58gProtein 5.94g

35. Chaffle Fruit Snacks

Preparation time: 10 minutes

Cooking Time: 14 Minutes

Servings: 2

Ingredients:

- 1 egg, beaten
- ½ cup finely grated cheddar cheese
- ½ cup Greek yogurt for topping
- 8 raspberries and blackberries for topping

Directions:

1. Preheat the waffle iron.
2. Mix the egg and cheddar cheese in a medium bowl.
3. Open the iron and add half of the mixture. Close and cook until crispy, 7 minutes.
4. Remove the chaffle onto a plate and make another with the remaining mixture.
5. Cut each chaffle into wedges and arrange on a plate.
6. Top each waffle with a tablespoon of yogurt and then two berries.
7. Serve afterward.

Nutrition: Calories 207Fats 15.29gCarbs 4.36gNet Carbs 3.gProtein 12.91g

36. Open-faced Ham & Green Bell Pepper Chaffle Sandwich

Preparation time: 10 minutes

Cooking Time: 10 Minutes

Servings: 2

Ingredients:

- 2 slices ham

- Cooking spray

- 1 green bell pepper, sliced into strips

- 2 slices cheese

- 1 tablespoon black olives, pitted and sliced

- 2 basic chaffles

Directions:

1. Cook the ham in a pan coated with oil over medium heat.

2. Next, cook the bell pepper.

3. Assemble the open-faced sandwich by topping each chaffle with ham and cheese, bell pepper and olives.

4. Toast in the oven until the cheese has melted a little.

Nutrition: Calories 36 Total Fat 24.6g Saturated Fat 13.6g Cholesterol 91mg Sodium 1154mg Potassium

440mg Total Carbohydrate 8g Dietary Fiber 2.6g Protein 24.5g Total Sugars 6.3g

37. Taco Chaffle

Preparation time: 8 minutes

Cooking Time: 20 Minutes

Servings: 2

Ingredients:

- 1 tablespoon olive oil
- 1 lb. ground beef
- 1 teaspoon ground cumin
- 1 teaspoon chili powder
- ¼ teaspoon onion powder
- ½ teaspoon garlic powder
- Salt to taste
- 4 basic chaffles
- 1 cup cabbage, chopped
- 4 tablespoons salsa (sugar-free)

Directions:

1. Pour the olive oil into a pan over medium heat.
2. Add the ground beef.
3. Season with the salt and spices.
4. Cook until brown and crumbly.
5. Fold the chaffle to create a "taco shell".

6. Stuff each chaffle taco with cabbage.

7. Top with the ground beef and salsa.

Nutrition: Calories 255 Total Fat 10.9g Saturated Fat 3.2g Cholesterol 101mg Sodium 220mg Potassium 561mg Total Carbohydrate 3g Dietary Fiber 1g Protein 35.1g Total Sugars 1.3g

38. Christmas Morning Choco Chaffle Cake

Servings:8

Cooking Time:5minutes

Ingredients:

- 8 keto chocolate square chaffles
- 2 cups peanut butter
- 16 oz. raspberries

Directions:

1. Assemble chaffles in layers.
2. Spread peanut butter in each layer.
3. Top with raspberries.
4. Enjoy cake on Christmas morning with keto coffee!

Nutrition: Protein: 3% 1Kcal Fat: 94% 207 Kcal Carbohydrates: 3% 15 Kcal

39. Lt Chaffle Sandwich

Preparation time: 10 minutes

Cooking Time: 15 Minutes

Servings: 2

Ingredients:

- Cooking spray
- 4 slices bacon
- 1 tablespoon mayonnaise
- 4 basic chaffles
- 2 lettuce leaves
- 2 tomato slices

Directions:

1. Coat your pan with foil and place it over medium heat.
2. Cook the bacon until golden and crispy.
3. Spread mayo on top of the chaffle.
4. Top with the lettuce, bacon and tomato.
5. Top with another chaffle.

Nutrition: Calories 238 Total Fat 18.4g Saturated Fat 5. Cholesterol 44mg Sodium 931mg Potassium 258mg Total Carbohydrate 3g Dietary Fiber 0.2g Protein 14.3g Total Sugars 0.9g

40. Mozzarella Peanut Butter Chaffle

Preparation time: 10 minutes

Cooking Time: 15 Minutes

Servings: 2

Ingredients:

- 1 egg, lightly beaten
- 2 tbsp peanut butter
- 2 tbsp Swerve
- 1/2 cup mozzarella cheese, shredded

Directions:

1. Preheat your waffle maker.
2. In a bowl, mix egg, cheese, Swerve, and peanut butter until well combined.
3. Spray waffle maker with cooking spray.
4. Pour half batter in the hot waffle maker and cook for minutes or until golden brown. Repeat with the remaining batter.
5. Serve and enjoy.

Nutrition: Calories 150Fat 11.5 carbohydrates 5.gSugar 1.7 protein 8.8 cholesterol 86 mg

DESSERT CHAFFLES

41. <u>Keto Smores Chaffle</u>

Preparation Time: 5 minutes

Cooking Time: 10 minutes

Servings: 2

Ingredients:

- One large Egg

- ½ c. Mozzarella cheese shredded

- ½ tsp Vanilla extract

- Two tbs swerve brown

- ½ tbs Psyllium Husk Powder optional

- ¼ tsp Baking Powder

- Pinch of pink salt

- ¼ Lily's Original Dark Chocolate Bar

- Two tbs Keto Marshmallow Creme Fluff Recipe

Directions:

1. Make the batch of Keto Marshmallow Creme Fluff.

2. Whisk the egg until creamy.

3. Add vanilla and Swerve Brown, mix well.

4. Mix in the shredded cheese and blend.

5. Then add Psyllium Husk Powder, baking powder, and salt.

6. Mix until well incorporated, let the batter rest 3-4 minutes.

7. Prep/plug in your waffle maker to preheat.

8. Spread ½ batter on the waffle maker and cook 3-4 minutes.

9. Remove and set on a cooling rack.

10. Cook second half of batter same, then remove to cool.

11. Once cool, assemble the chaffless with the marshmallow fluff and chocolate:

12. Using two tbs marshmallow and ¼ bar of Lily's Chocolate.

13. Eat as is, or toast for a melty and gooey Smore sandwich!

Nutrition: Calories: 0 Cal Total Fat: 8.1 g Saturated Fat: 0 g Cholesterol: 111.2 mg Sodium: 1352.5 mg Total Carbs: 3.1 g Fiber: 0.2 g Sugar: 0.7 g Protein: 8.3 g

42. Birthday Cake Chaffle

Preparation Time: 10 minutes

Cooking Time: 12 minutes

Servings: 2

Ingredients:

- 1 egg (beaten)
- 2 tbsp almond flour
- 1 tbsp swerve sweetener
- ½ tsp cake batter extract
- ¼ tsp baking powder
- 1 tbsp heavy whipping cream
- 2 tbsp cream cheese
- ½ tsp vanilla extract
- ½ tsp cinnamon
- Frosting:
- 1 tbsp swerve
- ¼ cup heavy whipping cream
- ½ tsp vanilla extract

Directions:

1. Plug the waffle maker to preheat it and spray it with a non-stick spray.

2. In a mixing bowl, combine the cinnamon, almond flour, baking powder and swerve.

3. In another mixing bowl, whisk together the egg, vanilla, heavy cream, and cake batter extract.

4. Pour the flour mixture into the egg mixture and mix until the ingredients are well combined, and you have formed a smooth batter.

5. Pour an appropriate amount of the batter into the waffle maker and spread out the waffle maker to cover all the holes on the waffle maker.

6. Close the waffle maker and bake for about 3 minutes or according to your waffle maker's settings.

7. After the cooking cycle, use a silicone or plastic utensil to remove the chaffle from the waffle maker.

8. Repeat steps 5 to 7 until you have cooked all the batter into chaffless.

9. For the cream, whisk together the swerve, heavy cream and vanilla extract until smooth and fluffy.

10. To assemble the cake, place one chaffle on a flat surface and spread 1/3 of the cream over it. Layer another chaffle on the first one and spread 1/3 of the cream over it too. Repeat this for the last chaffle and the remaining cream.

11. Cut cake and serve.

Nutrition: Servings: 2 Amount per serving Calories 249 Daily Value Total Fat 23.1g 30% Saturated Fat 11.8g 59% Cholesterol 144mg 48% Sodium 75mg 3% Total Carbohydrate 6g 2% Dietary Fiber 1.1g 4% Total Sugars 0.8g Protein 5.8g Vitamin D 27mcg 136% Calcium 92mg 7% Iron 1mg 5% Potassium 139mg 3%

43. Strawberry Shortcake Chaffle

Preparation Time: 5 minutes

Cooking Time: 8 minutes

Servings: 2

Ingredients:

- ½ tsp cinnamon
- ½ cup shredded mozzarella cheese
- 1 tsp sugar free maple syrup
- 2 tsp granulated swerve
- 1 egg (beaten)
- 1 tbsp almond flour
- Topping:
- 3 fresh strawberries (sliced)
- 2 tsp granulated swerve
- 1 tbsp heavy cream
- ¼ tsp vanilla extract
- 4 tbsp cream cheese (softened)

Directions:

1. Plug the waffle maker to preheat it and spray it with a non-stick cooking spray.

2. In a mixing bowl, combine the cinnamon, swerve, cheese and almond flour. Add the egg and maple syrup. Mix until the ingredients are well combined.

3. Close the waffle maker and cook for about 4 minutes or according to your waffle maker's settings.

4. After the cooking cycle, remove the chaffle from the waffle maker with a plastic or silicone utensil.

5. Repeat steps 3 to 5 until you have cooked all the batter into chaffless.

6. For the topping, combine the cream cheese, swerve vanilla and heavy cream in a mixing bowl. Whisk until the mixture is smooth and fluffy.

7. Top the chaffless with the cream and sliced strawberries.

8. Serve and enjoy.

Nutrition: Servings: 2 Amount per serving Calories 180% Daily Value Total Fat 15g 19% Saturated Fat 7.7g 38% Cholesterol 118mg 39% Sodium 137mg 6% Total Carbohydrate 5.2g 2%

Dietary Fiber 1.1g 4% Total Sugars 1.3g Protein 7.3g Vitamin D 12mcg 58% Calcium 54mg 4% Iron 1mg 5% Potassium 90mg 2%

44. Carrot Cake Chaffle

Preparation Time: 10 minutes

Cooking Time: 18 minutes

Servings: 10 (6 mini chaffles)

Ingredients:

- 1 tbsp toasted pecans (chopped)
- 2 tbsp granulated swerve
- 1 tsp pumpkin spice
- 1 tsp baking powder
- ½ shredded carrots
- 2 tbsp butter (melted)
- 1 tsp cinnamon
- 1 tsp vanilla extract (optional)
- 2 tbsp heavy whipping cream
- ¾ cup almond flour
- 1 egg (beaten)
- Butter cream cheese frosting:
- ½ cup cream cheese (softened)
- ¼ cup butter (softened)
- ½ tsp vanilla extract
- ¼ cup granulated swerve

Directions:

1. Plug the chaffle maker to preheat it and spray it with a non-stick cooking spray.
2. In a mixing bowl, combine the almond flour, cinnamon, carrot, pumpkin spice and swerve.
3. In another mixing bowl, whisk together the eggs, butter, heavy whipping cream, and vanilla extract.
4. Pour the flour mixture into the egg mixture and mix until you form a smooth batter.
5. Fold in the chopped pecans.
6. Close the waffle maker and cook for about 3 minutes or according to your waffle maker's settings.
7. After the cooking cycle, use a plastic or silicone utensil to remove the chaffle from the waffle maker.
8. Repeat steps 6 to 8 until you have cooked all the batter into chaffless.
9. For the frosting, combine the cream cheese and cutter int a mixer and mix until well combined.
10. Add the swerve and vanilla extract and slowly until the sweetener is well incorporated. Mix on high until the frosting is fluffy.

11. Place one chaffle on a flat surface and spread some cream frosting over it. Layer another chaffle over the first one a spread some cream over it too.

12. Repeat step 12 until you have assembled all the chaffless into a cake.

13. Cut and serve.

Nutrition: Servings: 10 Amount per serving Calories 181 % Daily Value Total Fat 17.4g 22% Saturated Fat 8.1g 41% Cholesterol 52mg 17% Sodium 93mg 4% Total Carbohydrate 4.5g 2% Dietary Fiber 1.2g 4% Total Sugars 0.6g Protein 3.5g Vitamin D 8mcg 39% Calcium 61mg 5% Iron 1mg 4% Potassium 91mg 2%

45. <u>Chaffless with Keto Ice Cream</u>

Preparation Time: 10 minutes

Cooking Time: 14 minutes

Servings: 2

Ingredients:

- one egg, beaten
- ½ cup finely grated mozzarella cheese
- ¼ cup almond flour
- 2 tbsp Swerve confectioner's sugar
- 1/8 tsp xanthan gum
- Low-carb ice cream (flavor of your choice) for serving

Directions:

1. Preheat the waffle iron.
2. In a medium bowl, mix all the ingredients except the ice cream.
3. Open the iron and add half of the mixture. Close and cook until crispy, 7 minutes.
4. Transfer the chaffle to a plate and make the second one with the remaining batter.
5. On each chaffle, add a scoop of low carb ice cream, fold into half-moons and enjoy.

Nutrition: Calories: 89 Cal Total Fat: 6.48 g Saturated Fat: 0 g Cholesterol: 0 mg Sodium: 0 mg Total Carbs: 1.37 g Fibre: 0 g Sugar: 0 g Protein: 5.91 g

SNACKS AND APPETIZER CHAFFLES

46. Chaffle Tacos

Preparation Time: 10 minutes

Cooking Time: 15 minutes

Servings: 4

Ingredients:

- Chaffle:
- 2 tbsp coconut flour
- 3 eggs (beaten)
- ½ cup shredded mozzarella cheese
- ½ cup shredded cheddar cheese
- A pinch of salt
- ½ tsp oregano
- Taco Filling:
- 1 garlic clove (minced)
- 1 small onion (finely chopped)
- ½ pound ground beef

- 1 tsp olive oil
- 1 tsp cumin
- ½ tsp Italian seasoning
- 1 tsp paprika
- 1 tsp chili powder
- 1 roma tomato (diced)
- 1 green bell pepper (diced)
- 4 tbsp sour cream
- 1 tbsp chopped green onions

Directions:

1. . Plug the waffle maker to preheat it and spray it with a non-stick cooking spray.
2. In a mixing bowl, combine the mozzarella cheese, cheddar, coconut flour, salt, and oregano. Add the eggs and mix until the ingredients are well combined.
3. Fill the waffle maker with an appropriate amount of the batter. Spread the mixture to the edges to cover all the holes on the waffle maker.
4. Close the waffle maker and cook for about 5 minutes or according to the waffle maker's settings.
5. After the cooking cycle, use a plastic or silicone utensil to remove the chaffle from the waffle maker. Set aside.

6. Repeat steps 3 to 5 until you have cooked all the batter into chaffless.

7. Heat a large skillet over medium to high heat.

8. Transfer the beef to a paper towel-lined plate to drain and wipe the skillet clean.

9. Add the olive oil and leave it to get hot.

10. Add the onions and garlic and saute for 3-4 minutes or until the onion is translucent, stirring often.

11. Add the diced tomatoes and green pepper—Cook for 1 minute.

12. Add the browned ground beef. Stir in the cumin, paprika, chilli powder, and Italian seasoning.

13. Reduce the heat and cook on low for about 8 minutes, often stirring to prevent burning.

14. Remove the skillet from heat.

15. Scoop the taco mixture into the chaffless and top with chopped green onion and sour cream.

16. Enjoy.

Nutrition: Servings: 4 Amount per serving Calories 321 % Daily Value Total Fat 17.5g 22% Saturated Fat 8.5g 43% Cholesterol 196mg 65% Sodium 266mg 12% Total Carbohydrate 12.6g 5% Dietary Fiber 4.4g 16% Total Sugars

4.5g Protein 28.6g Vitamin D 13mcg 66% Calcium 156mg 12% Iron 13mg 74% Potassium 533mg 11%

47. **Chicken Parmesan Chaffle**

Preparation Time: 5 minutes

Cooking Time: 13 minutes

Servings: 2

Ingredients:

- 1 egg (beaten)
- ½ cup shredded chicken
- 2 tbsp shredded parmesan cheese
- 1/3 cup shredded mozzarella cheese
- ¼ tsp garlic powder
- ¼ tsp onion powder
- 2 tbsp marinara sauce
- 1 tsp Italian seasoning
- Garnish:
- 1 tbsp chopped green onions

Directions:

1. Plug the waffle maker to preheat it and spray it with a non-stick cooking spray.
2. In a mixing bowl, combine the mozzarella cheese, shredded chicken, Italian seasoning, onion powder, and

garlic powder. Add the egg and mix until the ingredients are well combined.

3. Pour half of the batter into the waffle maker and spread out the mixture to the edges to cover all the holes on the waffle maker.

4. Close the waffle maker and cook for about 4 minutes or according to your waffle maker's settings.

5. Meanwhile, preheat your oven to 400°F and line a baking sheet with parchment paper.

6. After the cooking cycle, use a plastic or silicone utensil to remove the chaffle from the waffle maker.

7. Repeat 3, 4 and 6 to make the second chaffle.

8. Spread marinara sauce over the surface of both chaffless and sprinkle the parmesan cheese over the chaffless.

9. Arrange the chaffless into the baking sheet and place them in the oven—Bake for about 5 minutes or until the cheese melts.

10. Remove the chaffless from the oven and let them cool for a few minutes.

11. Serve and top with chopped green onion.

Nutrition: Servings: 2 Amount per serving Calories 144 % Daily Value Total Fat 6.7g 9% Saturated Fat 2.7g

14% Cholesterol   118mg   39% Sodium   212mg   9% Total Carbohydrate 3.7g 1% Dietary Fiber0.5g 2% Total Sugars 2g Protein   16.9g Vitamin   D   8mcg   39% Calcium   89mg 7% Iron 1mg 5%

Potassium 160mg 3%

48. **Broccoli and Cheese Chaffle**

Preparation Time: 5 minutes

Cooking Time: 15 minutes

Servings: 1

Ingredients:

- 1/3 cup broccoli (finely chopped)
- ½ tsp oregano
- 1/8 tsp salt or to taste
- 1/8 tsp ground black pepper or to taste'
- ½ tsp garlic powder
- ½ tsp onion powder
- 1 egg (beaten)
- 4 tbsp shredded cheddar cheese

Directions:

1. Plug the waffle maker to preheat it and spray it with a non-stick cooking spray.
2. In a mixing bowl, combine the cheese, oregano, pepper, garlic, salt, and onion. Add the egg and mix until the ingredients are well combined.
3. Fold in the chopped broccoli.

4. Pour an appropriate amount of the batter into your waffle maker and spread out the mixture to the edges to cover all the holes on the waffle maker.

5. Cook time may vary in some waffle makers.

6. After the cooking cycle, use a silicone or plastic utensil to remove the chaffle from the waffle maker.

7. Repeat steps 4 to 6 until you have cooked all the batter into chaffless.

8. Serve and top with sour cream as desired.

Nutrition: Servings: 1 Amount per serving Calories 198% Daily Value Total Fat 13.9g 18% Saturated Fat 7.3g 37% Cholesterol 193mg 64% Sodium 539mg 23% Total Carbohydrate 5.2g 2% Dietary Fiber 1.3g 5% Total Sugars 1.8g Protein 13.9g Vitamin D 19mcg 94% Calcium 259mg 20% Iron 2mg 10%

Potassium 222mg 5%

49. Simple Cornbread Chaffle

Preparation Time: 4 minutes

Cooking Time: 10 minutes

Servings: 4

Ingredients:

- 4 eggs
- 1 cup cheddar cheese, shredded
- 8 slices jalapeno, optional
- 1 tsp red hot sauce
- ¼ tsp low carb corn extract
- Pinch salt

Directions:

1. Preheat the waffle maker.
2. Crack the eggs in a small bowl and whip.
3. Add all the other ingredients and mix thoroughly.
4. Add a pinch of shredded cheese to the hot waffle maker. Cook for 30 seconds.
5. Pour half the egg mixture to the preheated waffle maker.
6. Cook for 5 minutes.
7. Remove, allow to cool, and enjoy.

Nutrition: Calories: 155 Cal Total Fat: 12 g Saturated Fat: 0 g Cholesterol: 0 mg Sodium: 0 mg Total Carbs: 1.2 g Fibre: 0 g Sugar: 0 g Protein: 10 g

50. <u>Tuna Chaffles</u>

Preparation Time: 5 minutes

Cooking Time: 8 minutes

Servings: 2

Ingredients:

- one packet Tuna, drained
- ½ cup mozzarella cheese
- One egg
- A pinch of salt

Directions:

1. Preheat, the waffle maker
2. Whip the egg in a small mixing bowl.
3. Add the tuna, cheese, and season with the salt. Mix well.
4. For a crispy crust, add a teaspoon of shredded cheese to the waffle maker and cook for 30 seconds.
5. Pour half the mixture to the mini waffle maker and cook for 4 minutes.
6. Remove it and repeat the process with the remaining tuna chaffle mixture.
7. Once ready, remove and enjoy warm.

Nutrition: Calories: 650 Cal Total Fat: 39 g Saturated Fat: 0 g Cholesterol: 0 mg Sodium: 0 mg Total Carbs: 6 g Fibre: 0 g Sugar: 0 g Protein: 63 g

CONCLUSION

The most well-documented advantage of the keto diet is the rapid weight loss. Contrary to beliefs, many people describe a reduction in hunger. Not only that, ketones can also minimize acne, and even enhance cardioprotection and maintain nerve activity, either way, once you start buying avocado crates, especially if you have avocado crates problem , You can contact the doctor for their opinions and guidelines. obesity. Everyone's requirements are different, and they don't apply to you. This applies to most citizens. In addition to focusing on fat quality, you can also evaluate protein when choosing foods. In a keto diet, you only need moderate amounts of protein-about 20% of total calorie consumption can come from protein-and some nuts seem to be rich in protein.

From the perspective of minerals and vitamins, make sure to integrate fibrous fruits and vegetables (such as cabbage, broccoli, and cauliflower).

According to the person's situation, it takes about 2-4 days to enter ketosis (it is recommended that the carbohydrate is low enough). Likewise, the amount of carbohydrates required to achieve ketosis may vary from person to person. "The initial weight loss will be very rapid, but remember that most of it will be contained in glycogen (carbohydrates) and water. After that, due to insufficient calories and consumption of more fat as fuel, weight loss will be slow. "With the development of the expression, winning the game slowly and steadily is extremely effective for diet. You can lose weight easily with ketones, but you may need to stay vigilant for a long time to help your body adapt to new eating habits.

Muffins can be frozen and processed, so a large portion can be made and stored for fast and extremely fast meals. If you don't have a waffle maker, just cook the mixture in a frying pan like pancakes and even cool it in a frying pan. They won't get all the fluffy aspects like using a waffle maker, but they will definitely be delicious. Depending on the cheese you choose, the number of carbohydrates and net calories may change a little. But, in general, whether you are using real full-fat cheese, the crunchy crust is completely carbohydrate-free. For up to a month, the husk will be frozen. However, defrosting absorbs a lot of water, which makes them difficult to crisp again. Boletus is rich in fat, moderate in protein content and low in carbohydrates. Chaffle is a very mature and popular technology that can fix people on ships. Compared to most forms of keto bread, this crusty bread is more durable and better. "You may want a high-carbohydrate diet. A non-stick waffle maker can make life easier, and it's a compromise choice, it's nice to embrace our happiness.

For everything transitioning to a lifestyle, please give yourself some time to adapt. You can see some rapid changes almost immediately, but to reduce the burden, even if the rate of improvement slows down, you must follow the plan. Slowing down does not mean that the new diet has stopped working. This simply means that the body is actually adjusting itself to adapt to the new eating habits. Things like losing weight or reducing unnecessary overweight are just a side effect of a healthy, better lifestyle that can support you in the long term (not only in the short term).

Lightning Source UK Ltd.
Milton Keynes UK
UKHW022007030521
383075UK00003B/339